WALL PILATES FOR WOMEN OVER 40

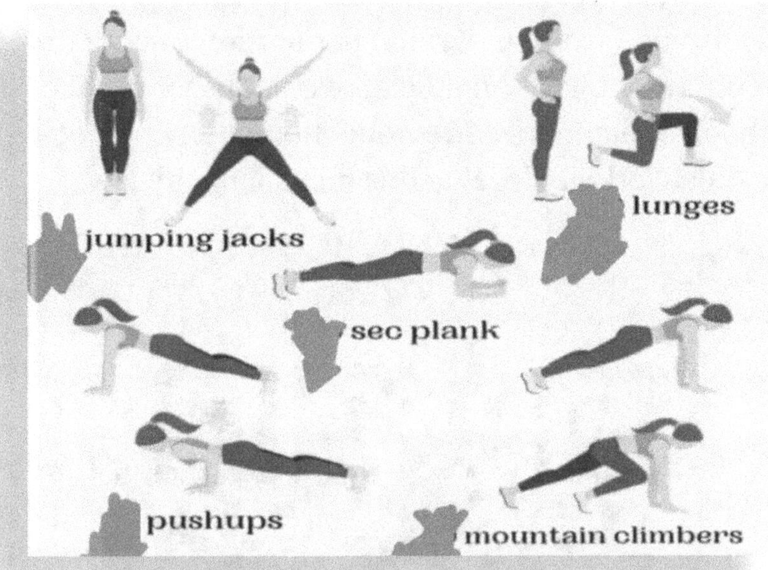

The complete 49 days body sculpting challenge to strengthen your muscles, tone your abs, glutes and improve your balance posture with step-by-step illustrated full body exercises.

CARLY EVELYN

SCAN TO GET MORE BOOKS BY THIS AUTHOR

IF YOU ARE STUCK, WHILE PRACTICING ANY OF THE EXERCISE IN THIS GUIDE, YOU CAN REACH THE AUTHOR AT TRAINERCCARLY@GMAIL.COM FOR GUIDANCE

TABLE OF CONTENT

INTRODUCTION

In the heart of a bustling city, amidst the concrete jungle and high-rise buildings, lived a woman named Maya. Maya was a dedicated Pilates enthusiast, and her quest for innovative ways to enhance her workouts led her to an unexpected discovery—the power of wall Pilates exercises.

One gloomy afternoon, Maya found herself feeling drained and demotivated. The monotony of her usual Pilates routine was taking its toll, and she longed for a fresh perspective. That's when a friend recommended trying wall Pilates, a technique she had recently stumbled upon.

Intrigued, Maya decided to give it a shot. She stood in front of her living room wall, ready to embark on a new fitness adventure. As she began, she immediately felt a connection between her body and the sturdy surface. The wall became her anchor, a source of stability that allowed her to explore a range of movements and engage muscles in ways she had never imagined.

Maya gracefully flowed from one exercise to another, seamlessly blending traditional Pilates with the newfound support of the wall. The vertical surface transformed into her training partner, enabling her to achieve perfect alignment, deeper stretches, and improved core engagement. The once-static wall now became a dynamic element in her workout routine.

Word of Maya's innovative approach to Pilates spread through her circle of friends and fitness enthusiasts. Inspired by her success, others eagerly embraced the wall Pilates trend. Maya's living room became a hub of creativity, where friends gathered to explore the countless possibilities, the wall offered.

Maya's journey didn't stop there. Her newfound passion for wall Pilates inspired her to organize community classes, introducing the innovative technique to a broader audience. Walls in gyms and fitness studios soon witnessed a surge in popularity, as people marveled at the transformative impact the humble wall could have on their Pilates practice.

As Maya continued to share her story and techniques through social media, she unintentionally sparked a global movement. Pilates enthusiasts from all corners of the world began incorporating wall exercises into their routines, creating a virtual community bound by a shared love for this unconventional approach.

Maya's story became synonymous with the fusion of tradition and innovation, proving that sometimes, all it takes to revitalize a passion is a fresh perspective and the support of a steadfast wall. In the end, Maya not only revitalized her own fitness journey but also left an indelible mark on the world of Pilates, showing that inspiration can emerge from the most unexpected places.

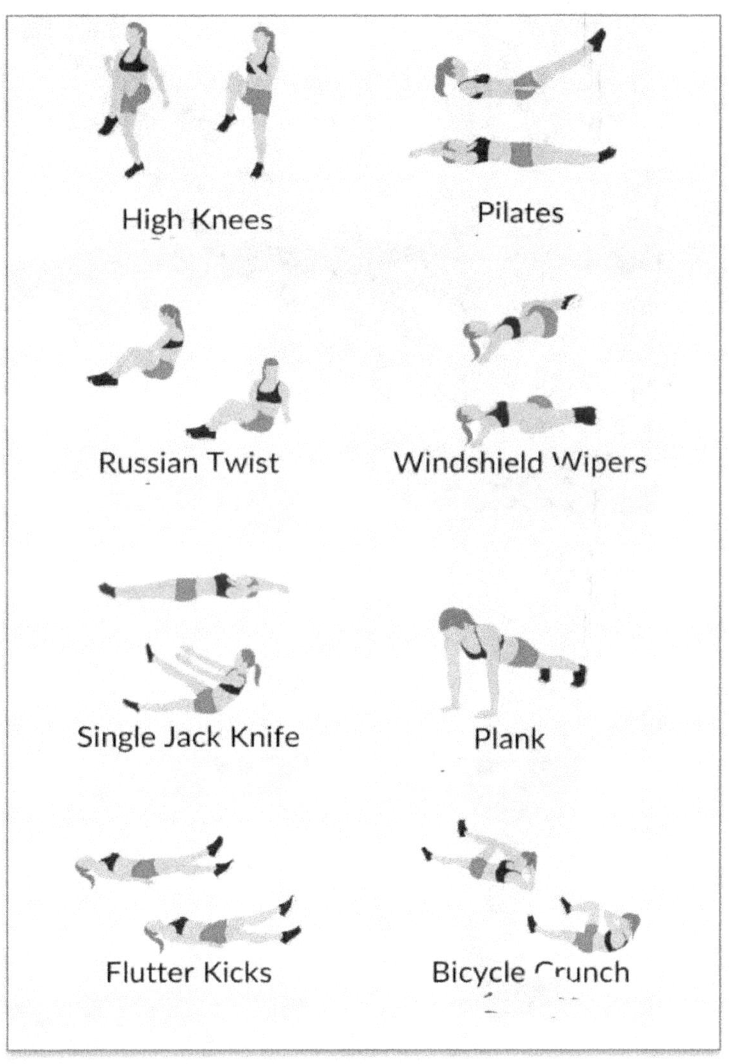

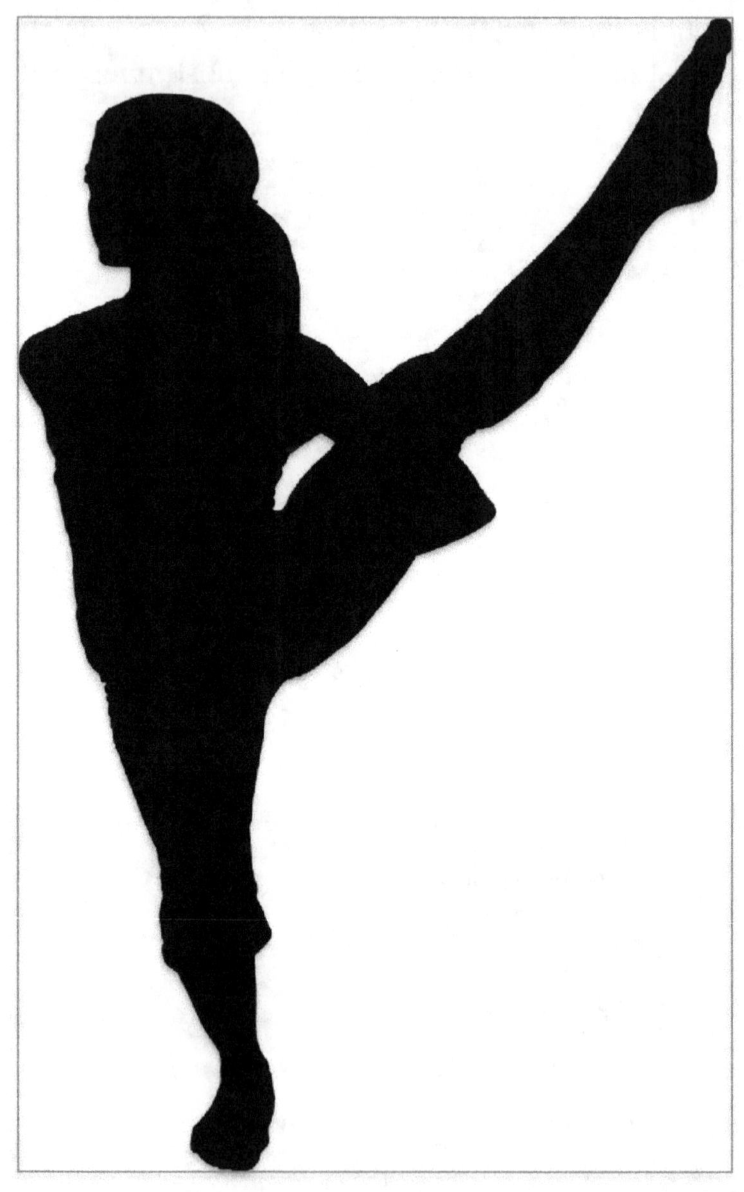

STEP BY STEP GUIDE WITH PICTURE ILLUSTRATION

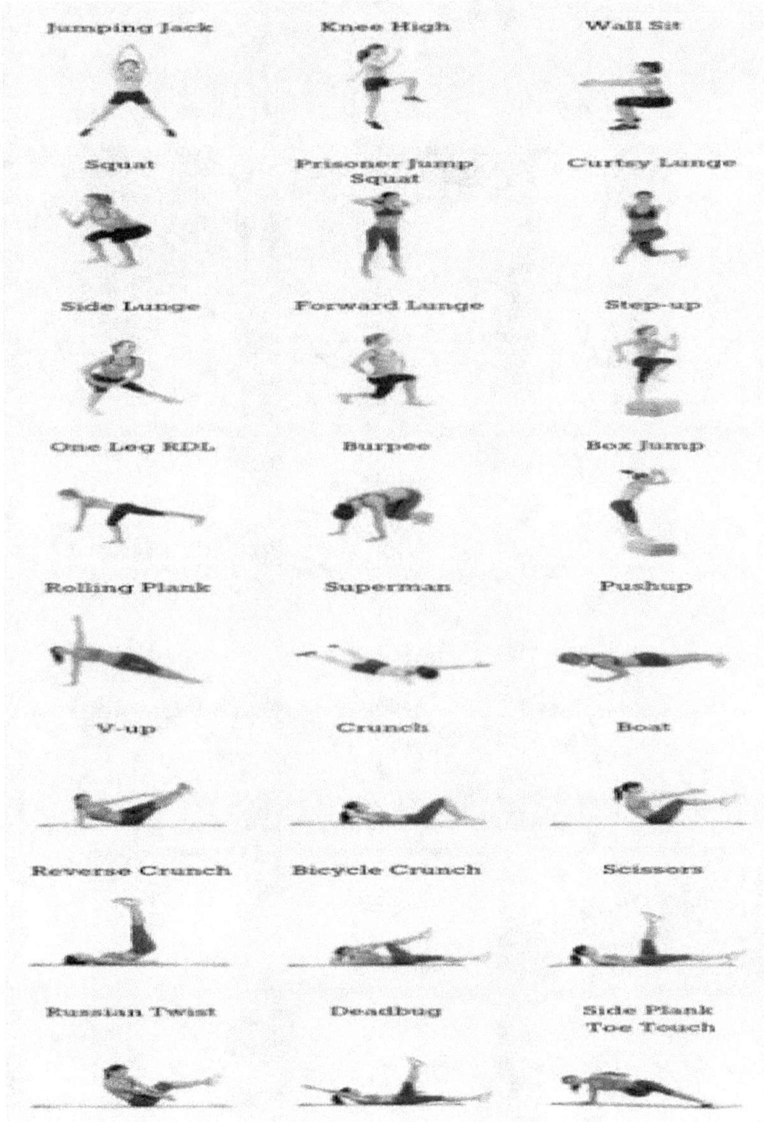

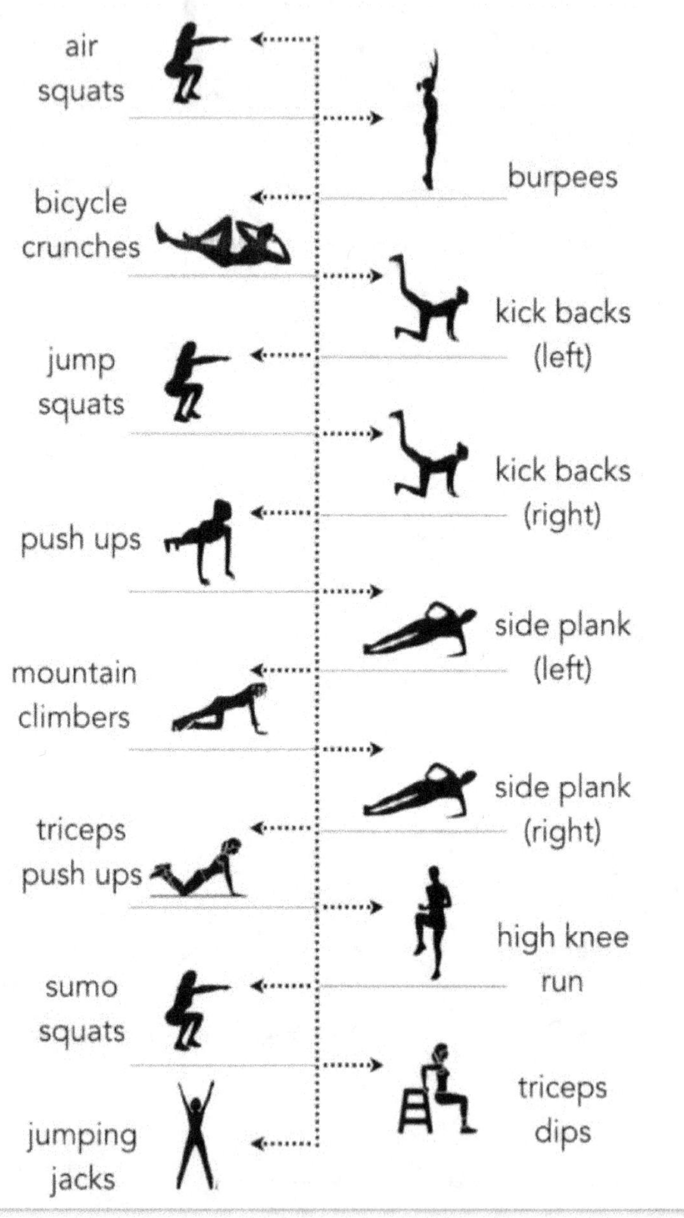
air
squats
burpees
bicycle
crunches
kick backs
(left)
jump
squats
kick backs
(right)
push ups
side plank
(left)
mountain
climbers
side plank
(right)
triceps
push ups
high knee
run
sumo
squats
triceps
dips
jumping
jacks

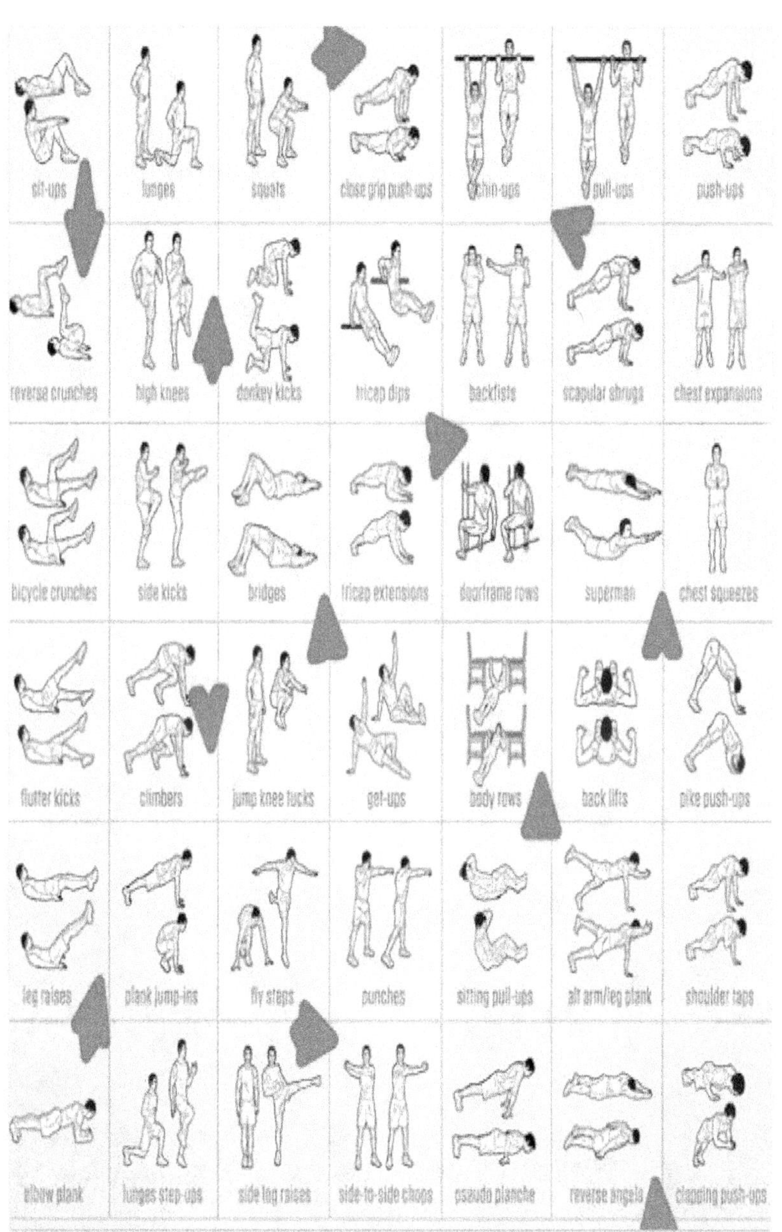

sit-ups
lunges
squats
close grip push-ups
chin-ups
pull-ups
push-ups
reverse crunches
high knees
donkey kicks
tricep dips
backfists
scapular shrugs
chest expansions
bicycle crunches
side kicks
bridges
tricep extensions
doorframe rows
superman
chest squeezes
flutter kicks
climbers
jump knee tucks
get-ups
body rows
back lifts
pike push-ups
leg raises
plank jump-ins
fly steps
punches
sitting pull-ups
alt arm/leg plank
shoulder taps
elbow plank
lunges step-ups
side leg raises
side-to-side chops
pseudo planche
reverse angels
clapping push-ups

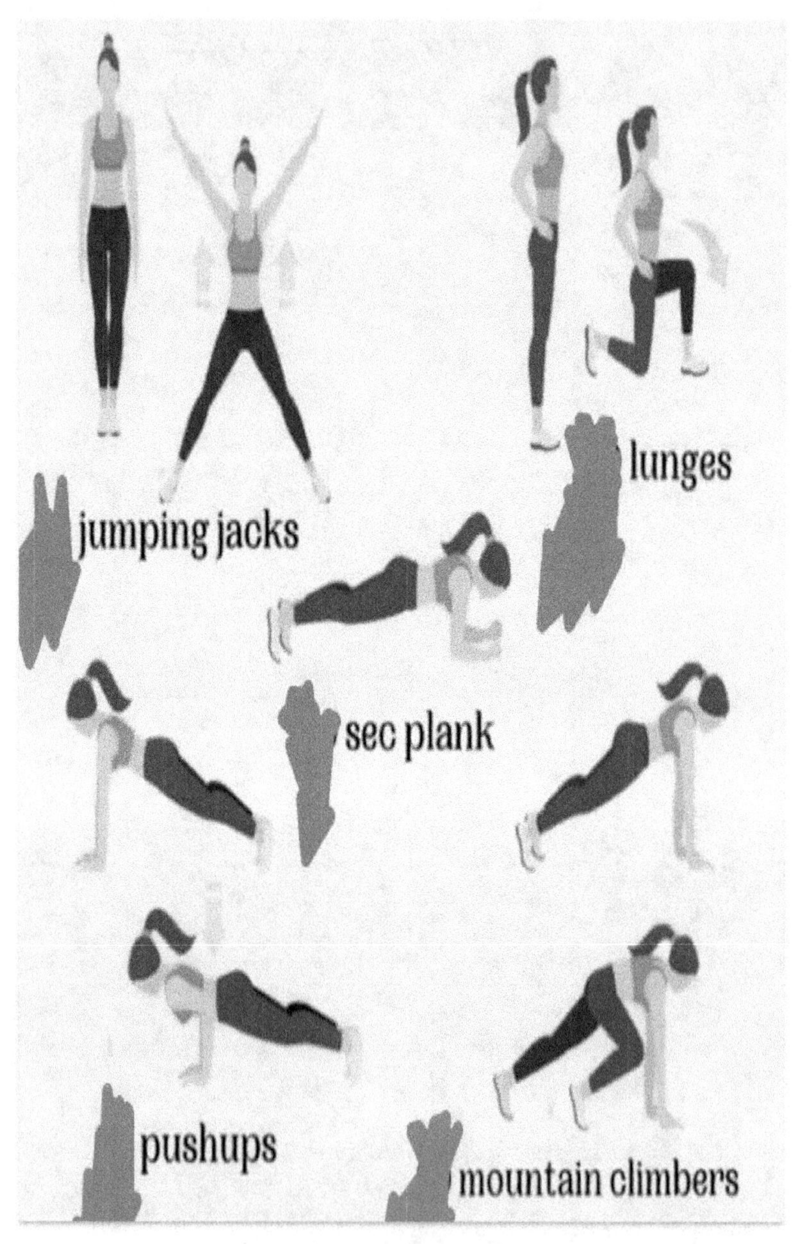
jumping jacks
lunges
sec plank
pushups
mountain climbers

It's vital to recognize that individual fitness requirements and capabilities differ. Before embarking on any new exercise routine, it is strongly advised to seek guidance from a fitness professional or healthcare provider. Moreover, the instructions provided are of a general nature and may necessitate adjustments based on your specific fitness level and any pre-existing health conditions.

40 WALL PILATES EXERCISES TAILORED FOR WOMEN OVER 40

1. Wall Squats:
   - Position yourself with your back against the wall.
   - Descend into a squat position, ensuring your back maintains contact with the wall.
   - Maintain the squat for 15-30 seconds before repeating.

2. Wall Sit with Leg Lifts:
   - Execute a wall sit.
   - Elevate one leg at a time, extending it straight in front of you.
   - Hold for a few seconds and alternate legs.

3. Wall Push-Ups:

- Stand facing the wall with arms extended.
- Execute push-ups by leaning towards the wall and then pushing back.

4. Wall Plank:

- Face the wall and place your hands against it.
- Retreat your feet until your body adopts a plank position.

5. Wall Bridge:

- Lie on your back with your feet pressed against the wall.
- Elevate your hips toward the ceiling.

6. Wall Crunches:

- Lie on your back with your feet positioned on the wall.
- Perform crunches by reaching towards your toes.

7. Wall Knee Tucks:

- Commence in a plank position facing away from the wall.
- Bring your knees towards your chest, engaging your core.

8. Wall Leg Raises:

- Lie on your back with your hands beneath your hips.

- Raise your legs towards the ceiling, maintaining their straight alignment.

9. Wall Side Plank:
- Lie on your side with your elbow directly under your shoulder.
- Elevate your hips to form a straight line from head to heels.

10. Wall Mountain Climbers:
- Assume a plank position facing the wall.
- Alternately draw your knees towards your chest.

11. Wall Lunge:
- Stand facing the wall, placing one foot behind you against the wall.
- Descend into a lunge position.

12. Wall Calf Raises:
- Face the wall with your hands upon it.
- Elevate your heels, lifting onto your toes.

13. Wall Side Leg Lifts:
- Lie on your side with your bottom leg against the wall.
- Elevate your top leg towards the ceiling.

14. Wall Scissor Kicks:
   - Lie on your back with your hands beneath your hips.
   - Elevate your legs and perform scissor-like movements.

15. Wall Roll Downs:
   - Stand facing the wall and descend, vertebra by vertebra.
   - Ascend back to the initial position.

16. Wall Toe Taps:
   - Lie on your back with legs raised towards the ceiling.
   - Lower one foot towards the wall, lightly tapping it.

17. Wall Bicycle Crunches:
   - Lie on your back with hands behind your head.
   - Bring one knee towards your chest while twisting to touch the opposite elbow.

18. Wall Chest Opener:
   - Stand facing the wall with arms extended.
   - Extend your arms to the sides, stretching your chest.

19. Wall Twist:
   - Sit on the floor facing the wall with bent knees.
   - Rotate your torso side to side, tapping the wall.

20. Wall Side Stretch:
   - Stand with your side facing the wall.
   - Extend your arm up and over, creating a side stretch.

21. Wall Chest Press:
   - Stand facing the wall with hands at chest height.
   - Push your hands into the wall, engaging your chest muscles.

22. Wall Leg Press:
   - Lie on your back with feet against the wall.
   - Press your feet into the wall, engaging your glutes and hamstrings.

23. Wall Triceps Dips:
   - Sit with your back against the wall and hands on the floor.
   - Lower your body into a dip, engaging your triceps.

24. Wall Hamstring Stretch:
   - Sit on the floor with one leg extended against the wall.
   - Reach forward to stretch your hamstring.

25. Wall V-Sit:
   - Sit on the floor facing the wall with legs lifted.

- Reach toward your toes, forming a V shape with your body.

26. Wall Oblique Crunches:
   - Lie on your back with feet on the wall.
   - Perform crunches, bringing your elbow to the opposite knee.

27. Wall Hip Flexor Stretch:
   - Kneel with one knee against the wall.
   - Lean forward to stretch your hip flexors.

28. Wall Plank with Knee Tuck:
   - Start in a plank position facing the wall.
   - Bring one knee toward your chest, alternating sides.

29. Wall Arm Circles:
   - Stand facing the wall with arms extended.
   - Circle your arms in both directions to engage your shoulders.

30. Wall Reverse Crunches:
   - Lie on your back with hands under your hips.
   - Lift your hips toward the ceiling, engaging your lower abs.

31. Wall Pike:
   - Start in a plank position facing away from the wall.

- Lift your hips toward the ceiling, forming an inverted V shape.

32. Wall W Stretch:
- Stand facing the wall with arms overhead.
- Form a W shape with your arms, opening your chest.

33. Wall Quadruped Leg Lifts:
- Kneel facing the wall with hands on the floor.
- Lift one leg toward the wall, keeping it straight.

34. Wall Side Plank with Leg Lift:
- Perform a side plank with your elbow on the floor.
- Lift your top leg toward the ceiling.

35. Wall Push-Up with Rotation:
- Perform a wall push-up.
- Rotate your torso, lifting one arm toward the ceiling.

36. Wall Butterfly Stretch:
- Sit facing the wall with the soles of your feet together.
- Gently press your knees toward the wall.

37. Wall Shoulder Bridge:
- Lie on your back with feet against the wall.
- Lift your hips toward the ceiling, engaging your glutes.

38. Wall Kneeling Leg Press:

   - Kneel facing the wall with one foot pressing against it.

   - Push your foot into the wall, engaging your quadriceps.

39. Wall High Knees:

   - Stand facing the wall.

   - Lift your knees toward your chest in a marching motion.

40. Wall Side Leg Press:

   - Lie on your side with your bottom leg against the wall.

   - Press your bottom leg into the wall, engaging your outer thigh.

These wall Pilates exercises provide a versatile range to target various muscle groups. Always warm up before starting, maintain proper form, and pay attention to your body. Modify exercises or seek guidance if you experience pain or discomfort. Embrace the benefits of this innovative Pilates approach and enjoy incorporating these movements into your fitness routine!

1. "Embark on a transformative odyssey of strength and poise through your wall Pilates practice."

2. "Grant empowerment to your physique, triumph over the wall – where Pilates serves as your artistic canvas."

3. "Transcend your boundaries, welcome the wall into your journey, and redefine the essence of your fortitude."

4. "Breathe in confidence, exhale doubt – such is the mastery of wall Pilates as an art form."

5. "Consider every wall as a bedrock for your resilience. Erect it, sculpt it, and assert your dominion."

6. "In the realm of wall Pilates: a juncture where strength converges with elegance, and determination harmonizes with grace."

7. "The wall stands as your pillar of support; your unwavering determination is the bedrock of your strength."

8. "Pilates transcends mere exercise; it is a pledge to the exceptional strength residing within you."

9. "Conquer not only the wall but also the apprehensions within you; unveil the undiscovered power that lies beneath."

10. "Regard your body as a masterpiece; let wall Pilates be the artisan's brush that sculpts and refines it."

11. "Seek equilibrium, embrace the wall, and radiate strength from the very core of your being."

12. "Wall Pilates: where the inconceivable transforms into 'I'm possible.'"

13. "Erect yourself, press against the wall, and acquaint yourself with a strength you never fathomed existed."

14. "In the realm of Pilates, your body serves as the canvas, and the wall emerges as your magnum opus."

15. "The wall is not a hindrance; it's an expansive canvas where your strength unfurls its narrative."

16. "Pilates: A testament to the foundation and resilience every woman deserves, fostering a spirit of flexibility."

17. "Conquer the formidable wall, embrace the fervor, and let your strength radiate luminously."

18. "Let the wall function as your reflective surface, mirroring the formidable strength you are evolving into."

19. "Engage in wall Pilates: where each challenge metamorphoses into an opportunity to showcase your inherent strength."

20. "Your strength is a distinctive signature; inscribe it onto the wall canvas through the practice of Pilates."

21. "The wall becomes your confidant, Pilates your expedition – a collaborative endeavor sculpting resilience."

22. "Pilates is not just a workout; it's a strategic investment in the prodigious power embedded within you."

23. "Stand resolute against the wall, stand firm in your might – Pilates bestows empowerment."

24. "Uncover the extraordinary within the ordinary – a mosaic painted one wall Pilates move at a time."

25. "Acknowledge the extraordinary capabilities of your body. Let the wall Pilates expedition commence."

26. "In wall Pilates, each movement is a stride towards a more robust, more empowered version of yourself."

27. "Embrace the wall, place trust in the process, and reveal the latent strength residing within."

28. "Pilates on the wall: Uplift your physique, elevate your cognition, and transcend into an elevated life."

29. "Your strength narrates a story uniquely yours. Etch it onto the wall with every deliberate Pilates movement."

30. "Pilates is not mere exercise; it's a festivity commemorating the remarkable woman you are metamorphosing into."

THANK YOU!!!

IF YOU FIND THIS BOOK TO BE INFORMATIVE, INSPIRING, OR SIMPLY ENJOYABLE, I WOULD BE IMMENSELY GRATEFUL IF YOU COULD SHARE YOUR THOUGHTS WITH OTHERS. YOUR HONEST REVIEW CAN MAKE A DIFFERENCE IN HELPING MORE INDIVIDUALS DISCOVER THE BENEFITS OF A NOURISHING AND MINDFUL APPROACH TO EATING. PLEASE CONSIDER LEAVING A REVIEW ON AMAZON AND SHARE YOUR EXPERIENCE.

THANK YOU ONCE AGAIN FOR CHOOSING THIS BOOK AS A COMPANION ON YOUR PATH TO A HEALTHIER, STRONGER, HAPPIER YOU.

CONCLUSION

In concluding this empowering journey through the world of wall Pilates exercises tailored for women, we've not only explored the physical dimensions of strength and flexibility but also delved into the profound connection between mind, body, and the resilient spirit within. Each exercise is a brushstroke, contributing to the masterpiece that is your holistic well-being.

As you navigate the pages of this book, envision the wall not as a barrier but as a canvas awaiting the vibrant strokes of your determination. Your body is a dynamic work of art, and wall Pilates serves as the medium through which you sculpt strength, grace, and unwavering confidence.

Now armed with a diverse repertoire of exercises, may you embark on your personal journey of transformation, breaking through perceived limits, and discovering the extraordinary within the ordinary. Let every movement be a celebration of your unique strength and a testament to the incredible woman you are becoming.

Don't forget, this is not just a book about exercises; it's a manifesto of empowerment, an invitation to embrace the wall, conquer challenges, and relish the exhilaration of your own strength. May each session be a step towards a more vibrant, resilient you—a living testament to the enduring power of perseverance, dedication, and the indomitable spirit of womanhood.

May the lessons learned within these pages resonate in your daily life, transcending the boundaries of the workout space. Your journey with wall Pilates is not just a temporary commitment; it's a lifelong partnership with your own potential.

As you close this book, envision yourself standing tall, confident, and transformed. The wall is no longer a hindrance; it's your ally, your canvas, and your partner in progress. Here's to the remarkable journey that lies ahead—a journey where strength meets elegance, determination meets grace, and every wall becomes a testament to the extraordinary woman you are. Embrace it. Own it. You are your masterpiece.

WALL PILATES WORKOUT PROGRESS

Weekly Workout Progress Tracker

WEEK OF THE MONTH: ___________

TYPE OF EXERCISE:	MUSCLE GROUP:	REPS:	S M T W T F S
__________________	_______________	_______	O O O O O O O
TYPE OF EXERCISE:	MUSCLE GROUP:	REPS:	S M T W T F S
__________________	_______________	_______	O O O O O O O
TYPE OF EXERCISE:	MUSCLE GROUP:	REPS:	S M T W T F S
__________________	_______________	_______	O O O O O O O
TYPE OF EXERCISE:	MUSCLE GROUP:	REPS:	S M T W T F S
__________________	_______________	_______	O O O O O O O
TYPE OF EXERCISE:	MUSCLE GROUP:	REPS:	S M T W T F S
__________________	_______________	_______	O O O O O O O
TYPE OF EXERCISE:	MUSCLE GROUP:	REPS:	S M T W T F S
__________________	_______________	_______	O O O O O O O
TYPE OF EXERCISE:	MUSCLE GROUP:	REPS:	S M T W T F S
__________________	_______________	_______	O O O O O O O

WHAT I LIKED ABOUT THIS WORKOUT:

WHAT I WILL CHANGE FOR NEXT WEEK:

WHAT I NOTICED WEEKLY ON MY BODY

WATER:

S M T W T F S

O O O O O O O

MEAL PLAN:

S M T W T F S

O O O O O O O

Weekly Workout Progress Tracker

WEEK OF THE MONTH: _______________

TYPE OF EXERCISE:	MUSCLE GROUP:	REPS:	S M T W T F S
			○○○○○○○
TYPE OF EXERCISE:	MUSCLE GROUP:	REPS:	S M T W T F S
			○○○○○○○
TYPE OF EXERCISE:	MUSCLE GROUP:	REPS:	S M T W T F S
			○○○○○○○
TYPE OF EXERCISE:	MUSCLE GROUP:	REPS:	S M T W T F S
			○○○○○○○
TYPE OF EXERCISE:	MUSCLE GROUP:	REPS:	S M T W T F S
			○○○○○○○
TYPE OF EXERCISE:	MUSCLE GROUP:	REPS:	S M T W T F S
			○○○○○○○
TYPE OF EXERCISE:	MUSCLE GROUP:	REPS:	S M T W T F S
			○○○○○○○

WHAT I LIKED ABOUT THIS WORKOUT:

WATER:

S M T W T F S

○○○○○○○

WHAT I WILL CHANGE FOR NEXT WEEK:

WHAT I NOTICED WEEKLY ON MY BODY

MEAL PLAN:

S M T W T F S

○○○○○○○

Weekly Workout Progress Tracker

WEEK OF THE MONTH: ___________

TYPE OF EXERCISE:	MUSCLE GROUP:	REPS:	S M T W T F S
___________	___________	______	O O O O O O O
TYPE OF EXERCISE:	MUSCLE GROUP:	REPS:	S M T W T F S
___________	___________	______	O O O O O O O
TYPE OF EXERCISE:	MUSCLE GROUP:	REPS:	S M T W T F S
___________	___________	______	O O O O O O O
TYPE OF EXERCISE:	MUSCLE GROUP:	REPS:	S M T W T F S
___________	___________	______	O O O O O O O
TYPE OF EXERCISE:	MUSCLE GROUP:	REPS:	S M T W T F S
___________	___________	______	O O O O O O O
TYPE OF EXERCISE:	MUSCLE GROUP:	REPS:	S M T W T F S
___________	___________	______	O O O O O O O
TYPE OF EXERCISE:	MUSCLE GROUP:	REPS:	S M T W T F S
___________	___________	______	O O O O O O O

WHAT I LIKED ABOUT THIS WORKOUT:

WATER:

S M T W T F S

O O O O O O O

WHAT I WILL CHANGE FOR NEXT WEEK:

WHAT I NOTICED WEEKLY ON MY BODY

MEAL PLAN:

S M T W T F S

O O O O O O O

Weekly Workout Progress Tracker

WEEK OF THE MONTH: _______________

TYPE OF EXERCISE:	MUSCLE GROUP:	REPS:	S M T W T F S
_______________	_______________	_______	ООООООО
TYPE OF EXERCISE:	MUSCLE GROUP:	REPS:	S M T W T F S
_______________	_______________	_______	ООООООО
TYPE OF EXERCISE:	MUSCLE GROUP:	REPS:	S M T W T F S
_______________	_______________	_______	ООООООО
TYPE OF EXERCISE:	MUSCLE GROUP:	REPS:	S M T W T F S
_______________	_______________	_______	ООООООО
TYPE OF EXERCISE:	MUSCLE GROUP:	REPS:	S M T W T F S
_______________	_______________	_______	ООООООО
TYPE OF EXERCISE:	MUSCLE GROUP:	REPS:	S M T W T F S
_______________	_______________	_______	ООООООО
TYPE OF EXERCISE:	MUSCLE GROUP:	REPS:	S M T W T F S
_______________	_______________	_______	ООООООО

WHAT I LIKED ABOUT THIS WORKOUT:

<u>WATER:</u>

S M T W T F S

ООООООО

WHAT I WILL CHANGE FOR NEXT WEEK:

WHAT I NOTICED WEEKLY ON MY BODY

<u>MEAL PLAN:</u>

S M T W T F S

ООООООО

Weekly Workout Progress Tracker

WEEK OF THE MONTH: _______________

TYPE OF EXERCISE:	MUSCLE GROUP:	REPS:	S M T W T F S
			○○○○○○○
TYPE OF EXERCISE:	MUSCLE GROUP:	REPS:	S M T W T F S
			○○○○○○○
TYPE OF EXERCISE:	MUSCLE GROUP:	REPS:	S M T W T F S
			○○○○○○○
TYPE OF EXERCISE:	MUSCLE GROUP:	REPS:	S M T W T F S
			○○○○○○○
TYPE OF EXERCISE:	MUSCLE GROUP:	REPS:	S M T W T F S
			○○○○○○○
TYPE OF EXERCISE:	MUSCLE GROUP:	REPS:	S M T W T F S
			○○○○○○○
TYPE OF EXERCISE:	MUSCLE GROUP:	REPS:	S M T W T F S
			○○○○○○○

WHAT I LIKED ABOUT THIS WORKOUT:

WATER:

S M T W T F S

○○○○○○○

WHAT I WILL CHANGE FOR NEXT WEEK:

WHAT I NOTICED WEEKLY ON MY BODY

MEAL PLAN:

S M T W T F S

○○○○○○○

Weekly Workout Progress Tracker

WEEK OF THE MONTH: _______________

TYPE OF EXERCISE: _______________ MUSCLE GROUP: _______________ REPS: _______ S M T W T F S ○○○○○○○

TYPE OF EXERCISE: _______________ MUSCLE GROUP: _______________ REPS: _______ S M T W T F S ○○○○○○○

TYPE OF EXERCISE: _______________ MUSCLE GROUP: _______________ REPS: _______ S M T W T F S ○○○○○○○

TYPE OF EXERCISE: _______________ MUSCLE GROUP: _______________ REPS: _______ S M T W T F S ○○○○○○○

TYPE OF EXERCISE: _______________ MUSCLE GROUP: _______________ REPS: _______ S M T W T F S ○○○○○○○

TYPE OF EXERCISE: _______________ MUSCLE GROUP: _______________ REPS: _______ S M T W T F S ○○○○○○○

TYPE OF EXERCISE: _______________ MUSCLE GROUP: _______________ REPS: _______ S M T W T F S ○○○○○○○

WHAT I LIKED ABOUT THIS WORKOUT:

WATER:

S M T W T F S
○○○○○○○

WHAT I WILL CHANGE FOR NEXT WEEK:

WHAT I NOTICED WEEKLY ON MY BODY

MEAL PLAN:

S M T W T F S
○○○○○○○

Weekly Workout Progress Tracker

WEEK OF THE MONTH: _______________

TYPE OF EXERCISE:	MUSCLE GROUP:	REPS:	S M T W T F S
_______________	_______________	_______	○○○○○○○
TYPE OF EXERCISE:	MUSCLE GROUP:	REPS:	S M T W T F S
_______________	_______________	_______	○○○○○○○
TYPE OF EXERCISE:	MUSCLE GROUP:	REPS:	S M T W T F S
_______________	_______________	_______	○○○○○○○
TYPE OF EXERCISE:	MUSCLE GROUP:	REPS:	S M T W T F S
_______________	_______________	_______	○○○○○○○
TYPE OF EXERCISE:	MUSCLE GROUP:	REPS:	S M T W T F S
_______________	_______________	_______	○○○○○○○
TYPE OF EXERCISE:	MUSCLE GROUP:	REPS:	S M T W T F S
_______________	_______________	_______	○○○○○○○
TYPE OF EXERCISE:	MUSCLE GROUP:	REPS:	S M T W T F S
_______________	_______________	_______	○○○○○○○

WHAT I LIKED ABOUT THIS WORKOUT:

WATER:

S M T W T F S
○○○○○○○

WHAT I WILL CHANGE FOR NEXT WEEK:

WHAT I NOTICED WEEKLY ON MY BODY

MEAL PLAN:

S M T W T F S
○○○○○○○

Weekly Workout Progress Tracker

WEEK OF THE MONTH: _______________

TYPE OF EXERCISE:	MUSCLE GROUP:	REPS:	S M T W T F S
			○○○○○○○
TYPE OF EXERCISE:	MUSCLE GROUP:	REPS:	S M T W T F S
			○○○○○○○
TYPE OF EXERCISE:	MUSCLE GROUP:	REPS:	S M T W T F S
			○○○○○○○
TYPE OF EXERCISE:	MUSCLE GROUP:	REPS:	S M T W T F S
			○○○○○○○
TYPE OF EXERCISE:	MUSCLE GROUP:	REPS:	S M T W T F S
			○○○○○○○
TYPE OF EXERCISE:	MUSCLE GROUP:	REPS:	S M T W T F S
			○○○○○○○
TYPE OF EXERCISE:	MUSCLE GROUP:	REPS:	S M T W T F S
			○○○○○○○

WHAT I LIKED ABOUT THIS WORKOUT:

WHAT I WILL CHANGE FOR NEXT WEEK:

WHAT I NOTICED WEEKLY ON MY BODY

<u>WATER:</u>

S M T W T F S

○○○○○○○

<u>MEAL PLAN:</u>

S M T W T F S

○○○○○○○

Weekly Workout Progress Tracker

WEEK OF THE MONTH: _______________

TYPE OF EXERCISE:	MUSCLE GROUP:	REPS:	S M T W T F S
			○○○○○○○
TYPE OF EXERCISE:	MUSCLE GROUP:	REPS:	S M T W T F S
			○○○○○○○
TYPE OF EXERCISE:	MUSCLE GROUP:	REPS:	S M T W T F S
			○○○○○○○
TYPE OF EXERCISE:	MUSCLE GROUP:	REPS:	S M T W T F S
			○○○○○○○
TYPE OF EXERCISE:	MUSCLE GROUP:	REPS:	S M T W T F S
			○○○○○○○
TYPE OF EXERCISE:	MUSCLE GROUP:	REPS:	S M T W T F S
			○○○○○○○
TYPE OF EXERCISE:	MUSCLE GROUP:	REPS:	S M T W T F S
			○○○○○○○

WHAT I LIKED ABOUT THIS WORKOUT:

WATER:

S M T W T F S
○○○○○○○

WHAT I WILL CHANGE FOR NEXT WEEK:

WHAT I NOTICED WEEKLY ON MY BODY

MEAL PLAN:

S M T W T F S
○○○○○○○

Weekly Workout Progress Tracker

WEEK OF THE MONTH: _______________

TYPE OF EXERCISE:	MUSCLE GROUP:	REPS:	S M T W T F S
_______________	_______________	_______	○○○○○○○
TYPE OF EXERCISE:	MUSCLE GROUP:	REPS:	S M T W T F S
_______________	_______________	_______	○○○○○○○
TYPE OF EXERCISE:	MUSCLE GROUP:	REPS:	S M T W T F S
_______________	_______________	_______	○○○○○○○
TYPE OF EXERCISE:	MUSCLE GROUP:	REPS:	S M T W T F S
_______________	_______________	_______	○○○○○○○
TYPE OF EXERCISE:	MUSCLE GROUP:	REPS:	S M T W T F S
_______________	_______________	_______	○○○○○○○
TYPE OF EXERCISE:	MUSCLE GROUP:	REPS:	S M T W T F S
_______________	_______________	_______	○○○○○○○
TYPE OF EXERCISE:	MUSCLE GROUP:	REPS:	S M T W T F S
_______________	_______________	_______	○○○○○○○

WHAT I LIKED ABOUT THIS WORKOUT:

WATER:

S M T W T F S
○○○○○○○

WHAT I WILL CHANGE FOR NEXT WEEK:

WHAT I NOTICED WEEKLY ON MY BODY

MEAL PLAN:

S M T W T F S
○○○○○○○

Weekly Workout Progress Tracker

WEEK OF THE MONTH: ___________________

TYPE OF EXERCISE:	MUSCLE GROUP:	REPS:	S M T W T F S
_________________	_________________	_______	○○○○○○○
TYPE OF EXERCISE:	MUSCLE GROUP:	REPS:	S M T W T F S
_________________	_________________	_______	○○○○○○○
TYPE OF EXERCISE:	MUSCLE GROUP:	REPS:	S M T W T F S
_________________	_________________	_______	○○○○○○○
TYPE OF EXERCISE:	MUSCLE GROUP:	REPS:	S M T W T F S
_________________	_________________	_______	○○○○○○○
TYPE OF EXERCISE:	MUSCLE GROUP:	REPS:	S M T W T F S
_________________	_________________	_______	○○○○○○○
TYPE OF EXERCISE:	MUSCLE GROUP:	REPS:	S M T W T F S
_________________	_________________	_______	○○○○○○○
TYPE OF EXERCISE:	MUSCLE GROUP:	REPS:	S M T W T F S
_________________	_________________	_______	○○○○○○○

WHAT I LIKED ABOUT THIS WORKOUT:

WHAT I WILL CHANGE FOR NEXT WEEK:

WHAT I NOTICED WEEKLY ON MY BODY

<u>WATER:</u>

S M T W T F S
○○○○○○○

<u>MEAL PLAN:</u>

S M T W T F S
○○○○○○○

Weekly Workout Progress Tracker

WEEK OF THE MONTH: ___________________

TYPE OF EXERCISE: MUSCLE GROUP: REPS: S M T W T F S
_______________   _______________   _______   ○○○○○○○

TYPE OF EXERCISE: MUSCLE GROUP: REPS: S M T W T F S
_______________   _______________   _______   ○○○○○○○

TYPE OF EXERCISE: MUSCLE GROUP: REPS: S M T W T F S
_______________   _______________   _______   ○○○○○○○

TYPE OF EXERCISE: MUSCLE GROUP: REPS: S M T W T F S
_______________   _______________   _______   ○○○○○○○

TYPE OF EXERCISE: MUSCLE GROUP: REPS: S M T W T F S
_______________   _______________   _______   ○○○○○○○

TYPE OF EXERCISE: MUSCLE GROUP: REPS: S M T W T F S
_______________   _______________   _______   ○○○○○○○

TYPE OF EXERCISE: MUSCLE GROUP: REPS: S M T W T F S
_______________   _______________   _______   ○○○○○○○

WHAT I LIKED ABOUT THIS WORKOUT:

WATER:

S M T W T F S
○○○○○○○

WHAT I WILL CHANGE FOR NEXT WEEK:

WHAT I NOTICED WEEKLY ON MY BODY

MEAL PLAN:

S M T W T F S
○○○○○○○

＃ *Weekly Workout Progress Tracker* WEEK OF THE MONTH: _______________

TYPE OF EXERCISE: MUSCLE GROUP: REPS: S M T W T F S

_______________   _______________   _______   ○○○○○○○

TYPE OF EXERCISE: MUSCLE GROUP: REPS: S M T W T F S

_______________   _______________   _______   ○○○○○○○

TYPE OF EXERCISE: MUSCLE GROUP: REPS: S M T W T F S

_______________   _______________   _______   ○○○○○○○

TYPE OF EXERCISE: MUSCLE GROUP: REPS: S M T W T F S

_______________   _______________   _______   ○○○○○○○

TYPE OF EXERCISE: MUSCLE GROUP: REPS: S M T W T F S

_______________   _______________   _______   ○○○○○○○

TYPE OF EXERCISE: MUSCLE GROUP: REPS: S M T W T F S

_______________   _______________   _______   ○○○○○○○

TYPE OF EXERCISE: MUSCLE GROUP: REPS: S M T W T F S

_______________   _______________   _______   ○○○○○○○

WHAT I LIKED ABOUT THIS WORKOUT:

WHAT I WILL CHANGE FOR NEXT WEEK:

WHAT I NOTICED WEEKLY ON MY BODY

<u>WATER:</u>

S M T W T F S

○○○○○○○

<u>MEAL PLAN:</u>

S M T W T F S

○○○○○○○

Weekly Workout Progress Tracker

WEEK OF THE MONTH: _______________

TYPE OF EXERCISE:	MUSCLE GROUP:	REPS:	S M T W T F S
_______________	_______________	_______	○○○○○○○
TYPE OF EXERCISE:	MUSCLE GROUP:	REPS:	S M T W T F S
_______________	_______________	_______	○○○○○○○
TYPE OF EXERCISE:	MUSCLE GROUP:	REPS:	S M T W T F S
_______________	_______________	_______	○○○○○○○
TYPE OF EXERCISE:	MUSCLE GROUP:	REPS:	S M T W T F S
_______________	_______________	_______	○○○○○○○
TYPE OF EXERCISE:	MUSCLE GROUP:	REPS:	S M T W T F S
_______________	_______________	_______	○○○○○○○
TYPE OF EXERCISE:	MUSCLE GROUP:	REPS:	S M T W T F S
_______________	_______________	_______	○○○○○○○
TYPE OF EXERCISE:	MUSCLE GROUP:	REPS:	S M T W T F S
_______________	_______________	_______	○○○○○○○

WHAT I LIKED ABOUT THIS WORKOUT:

WATER:

S M T W T F S

○○○○○○○

WHAT I WILL CHANGE FOR NEXT WEEK:

WHAT I NOTICED WEEKLY ON MY BODY

MEAL PLAN:

S M T W T F S

○○○○○○○